# FLOWER
## VOLUME 3.
### Mandala Adult Coloring Book

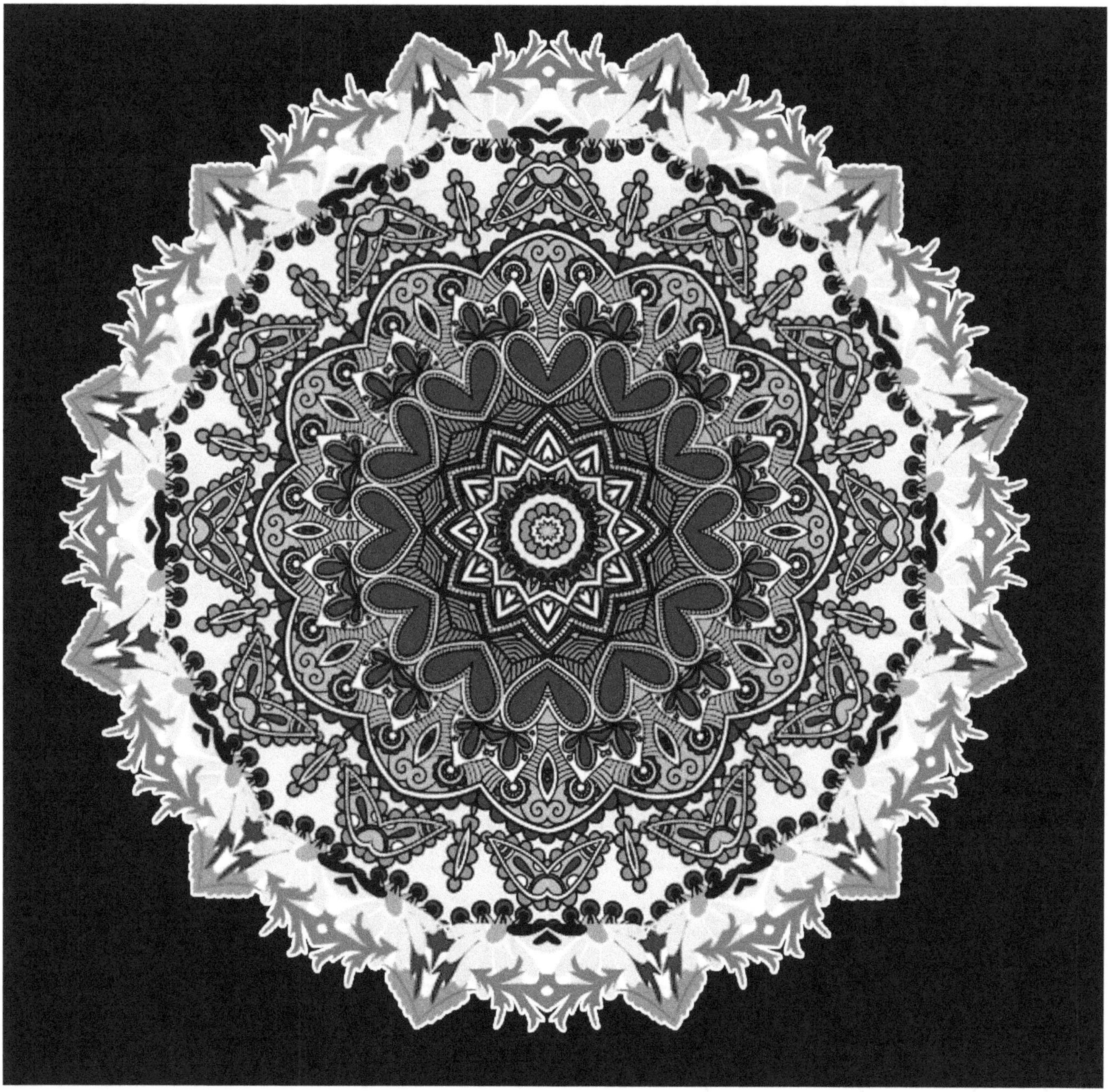

# COLOR TEST PAGE

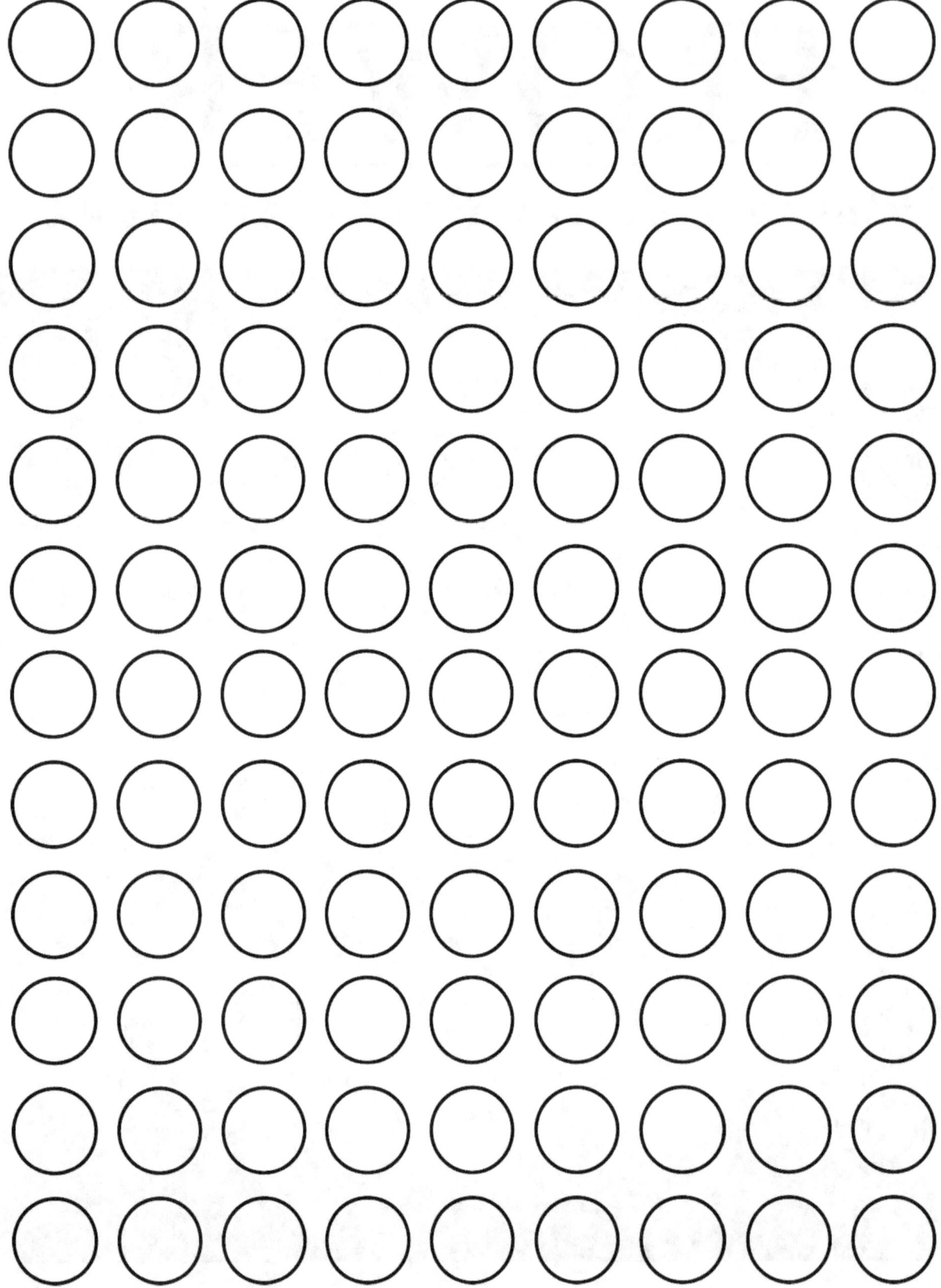

# COLOR TEST PAGE

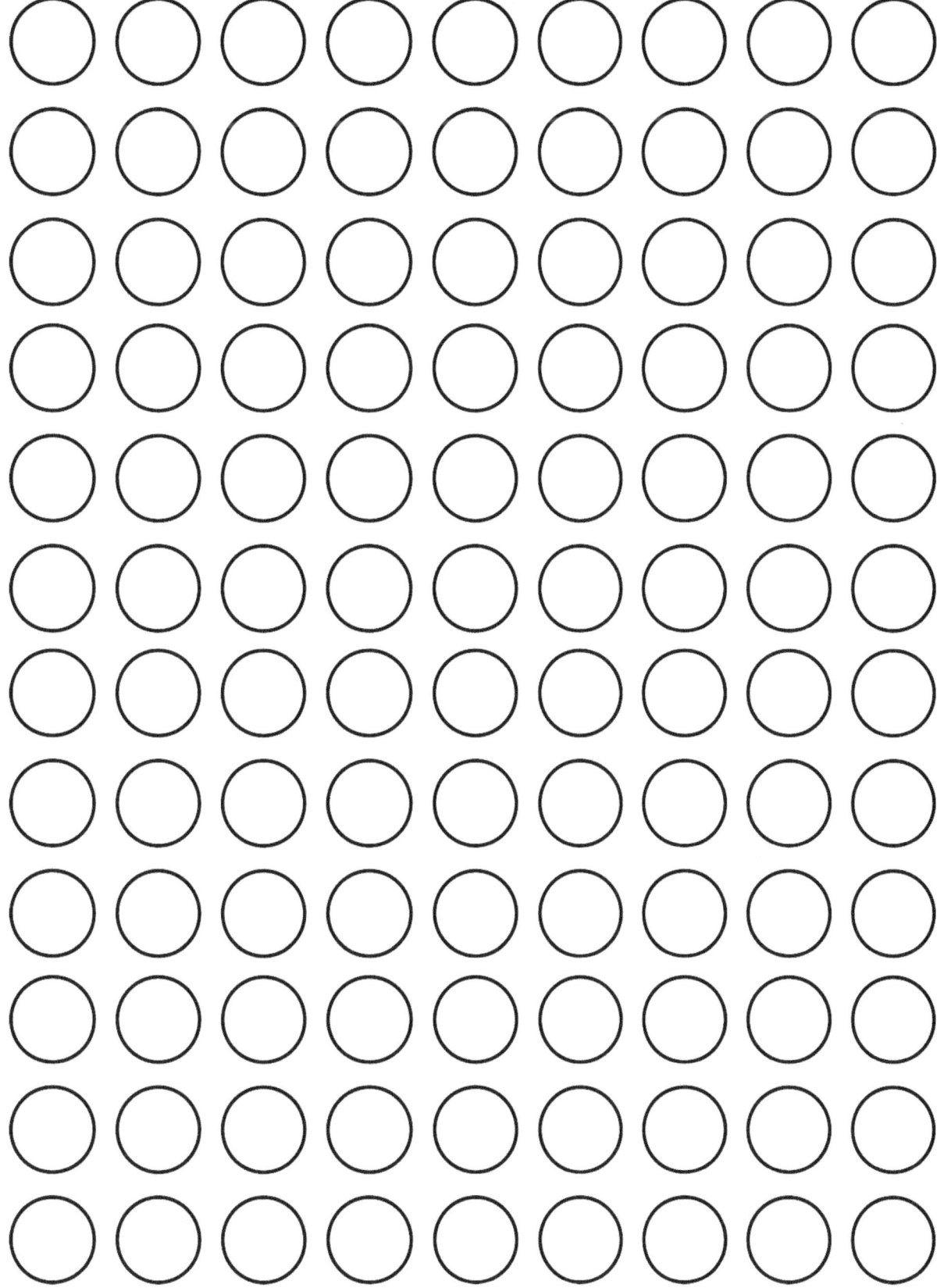

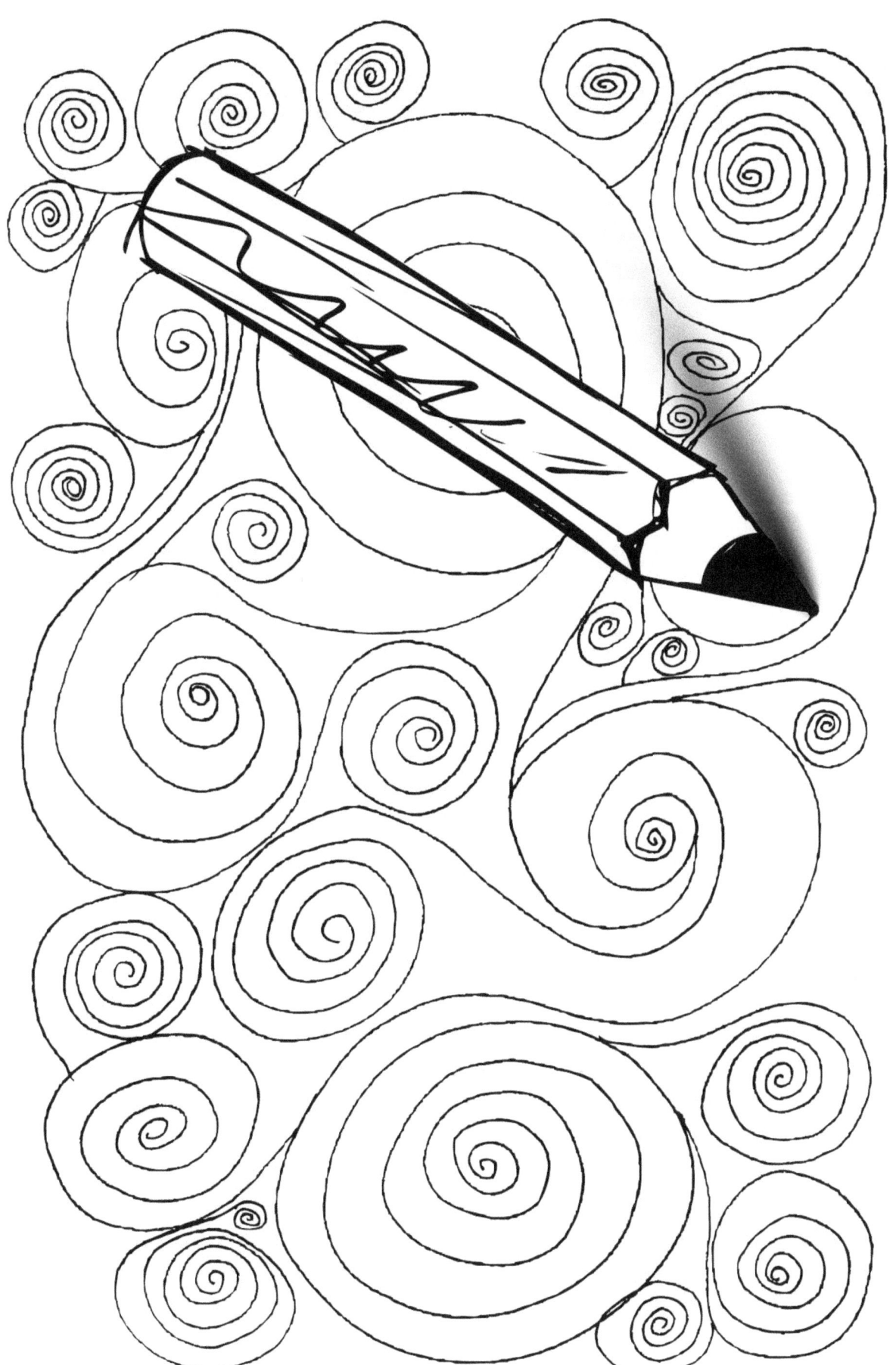

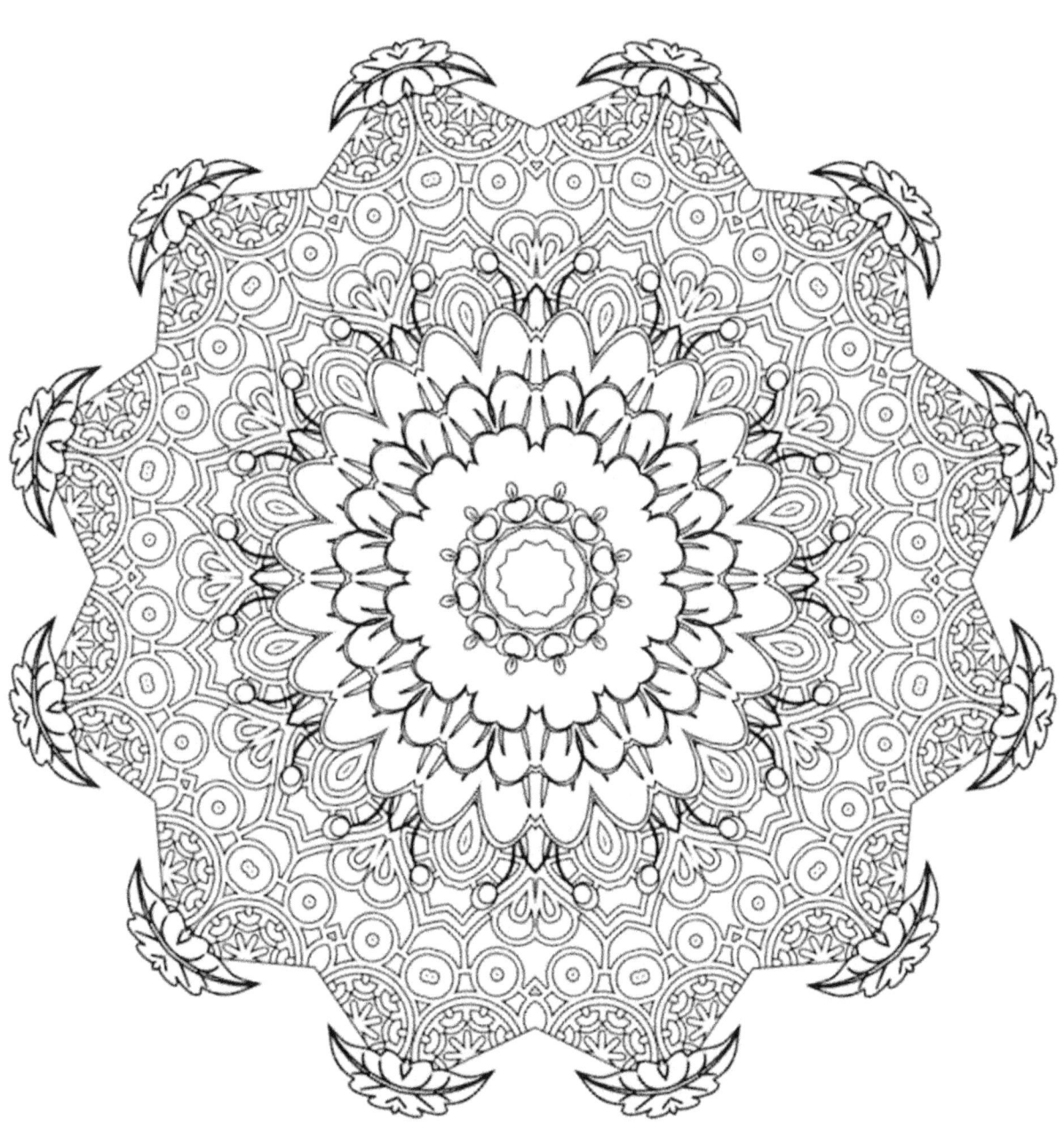

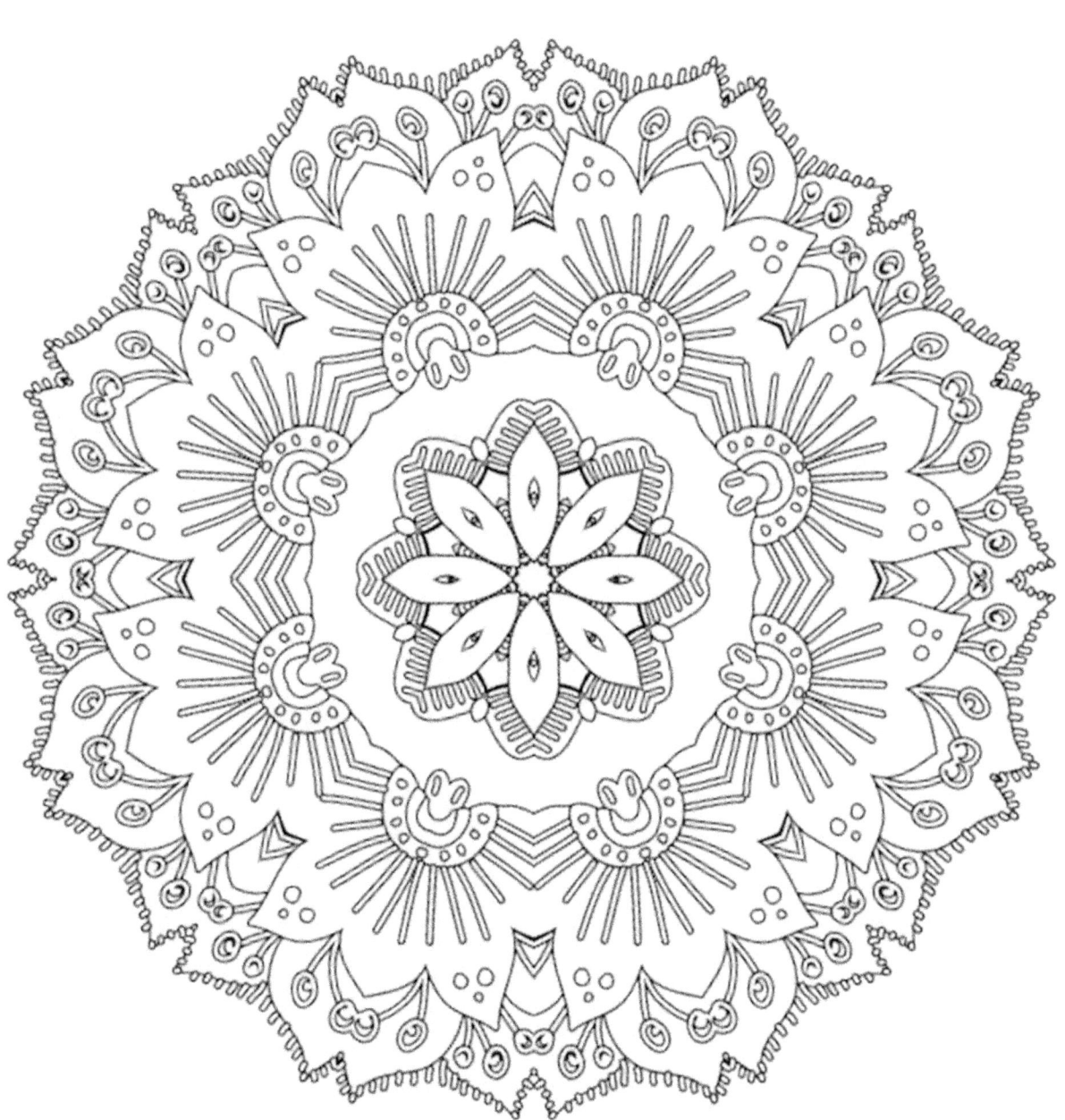

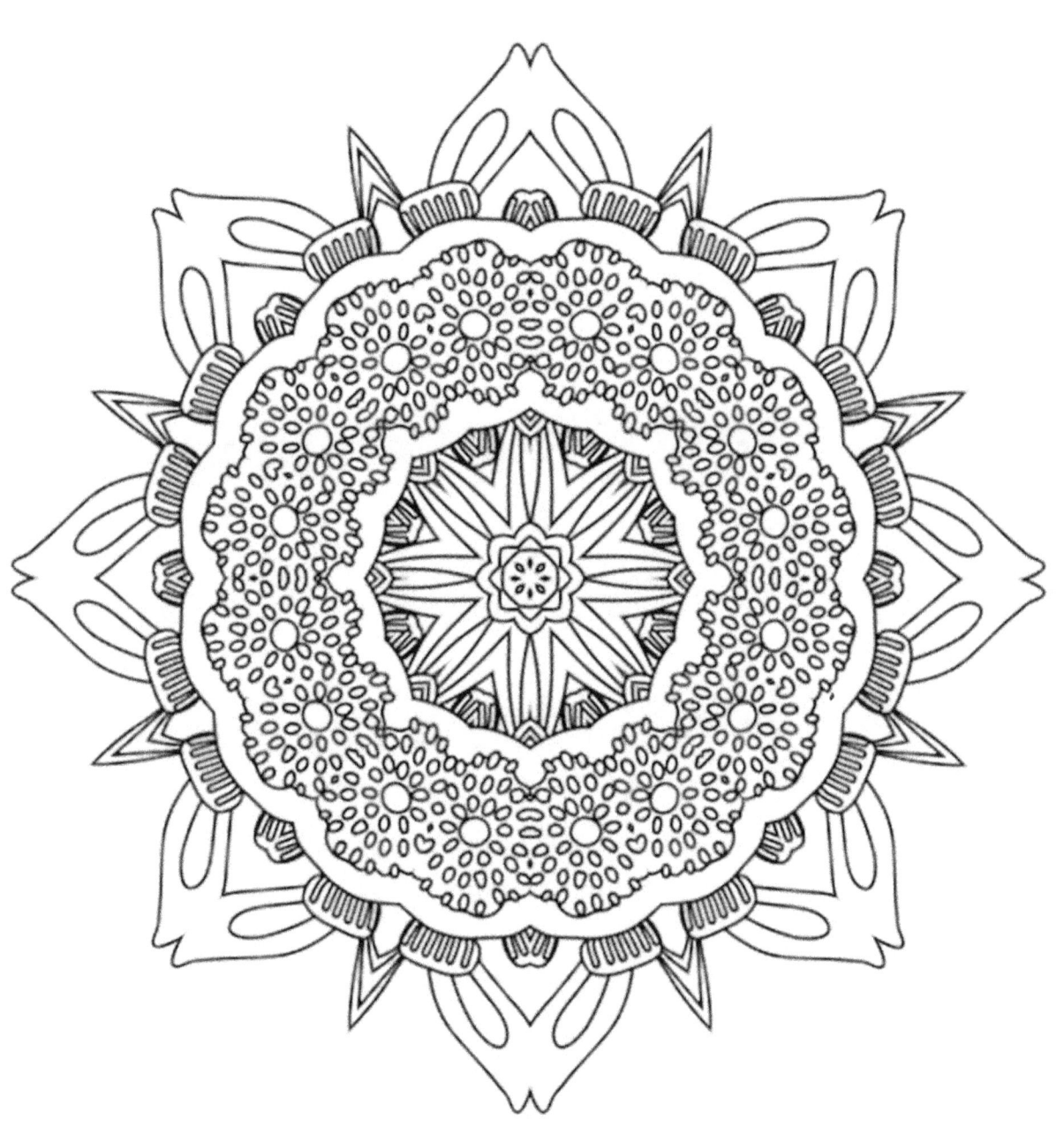

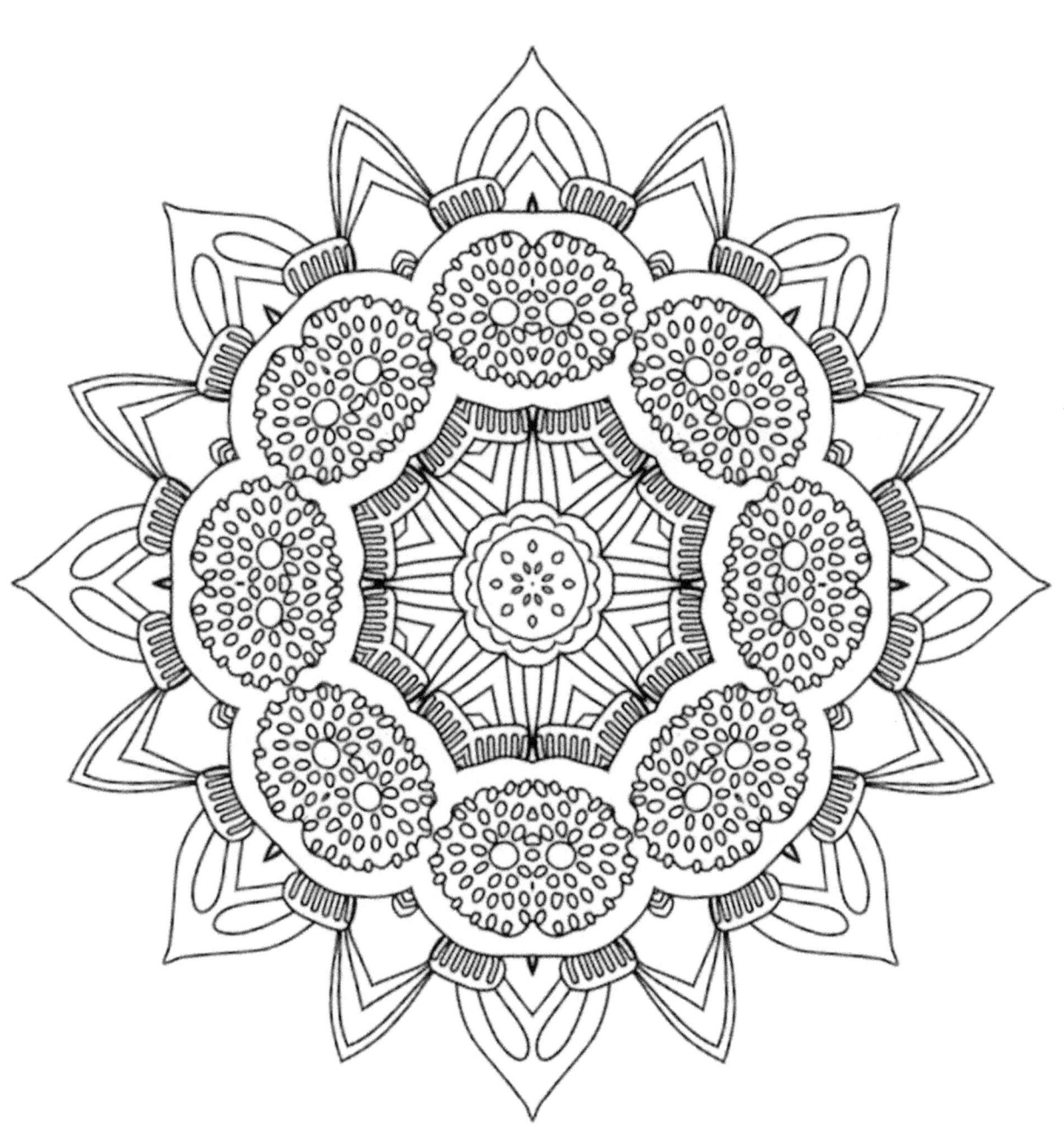

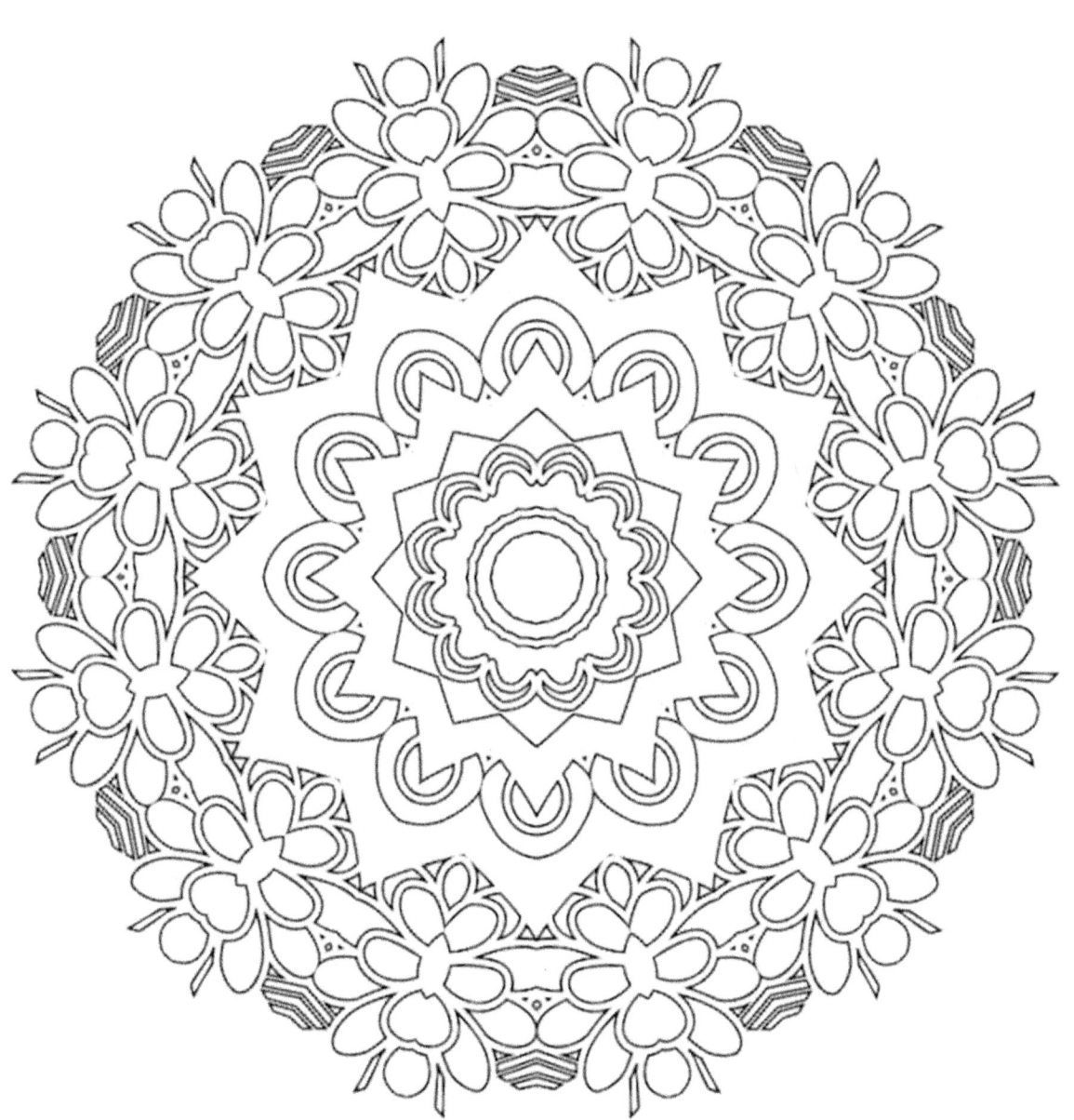

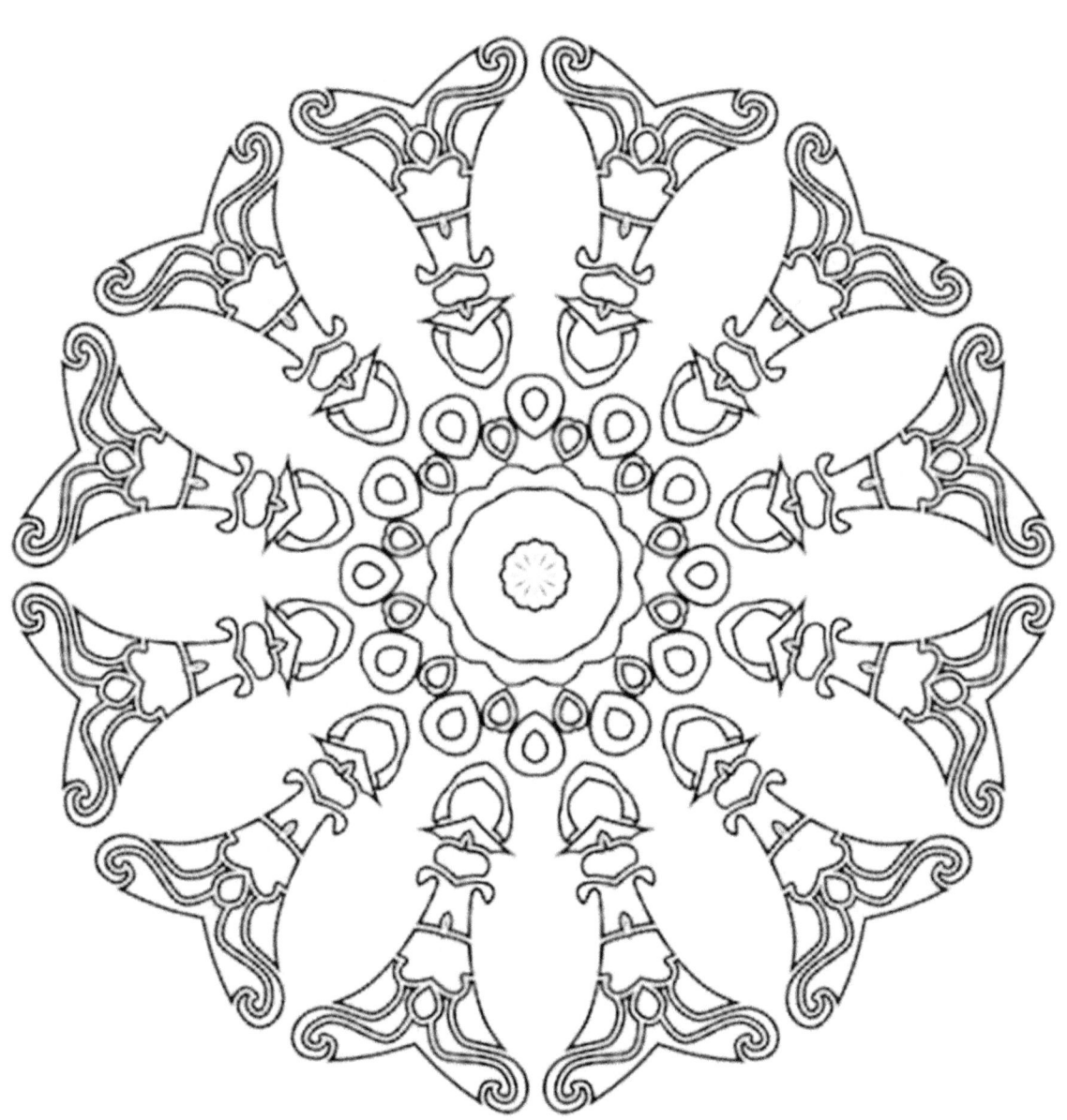

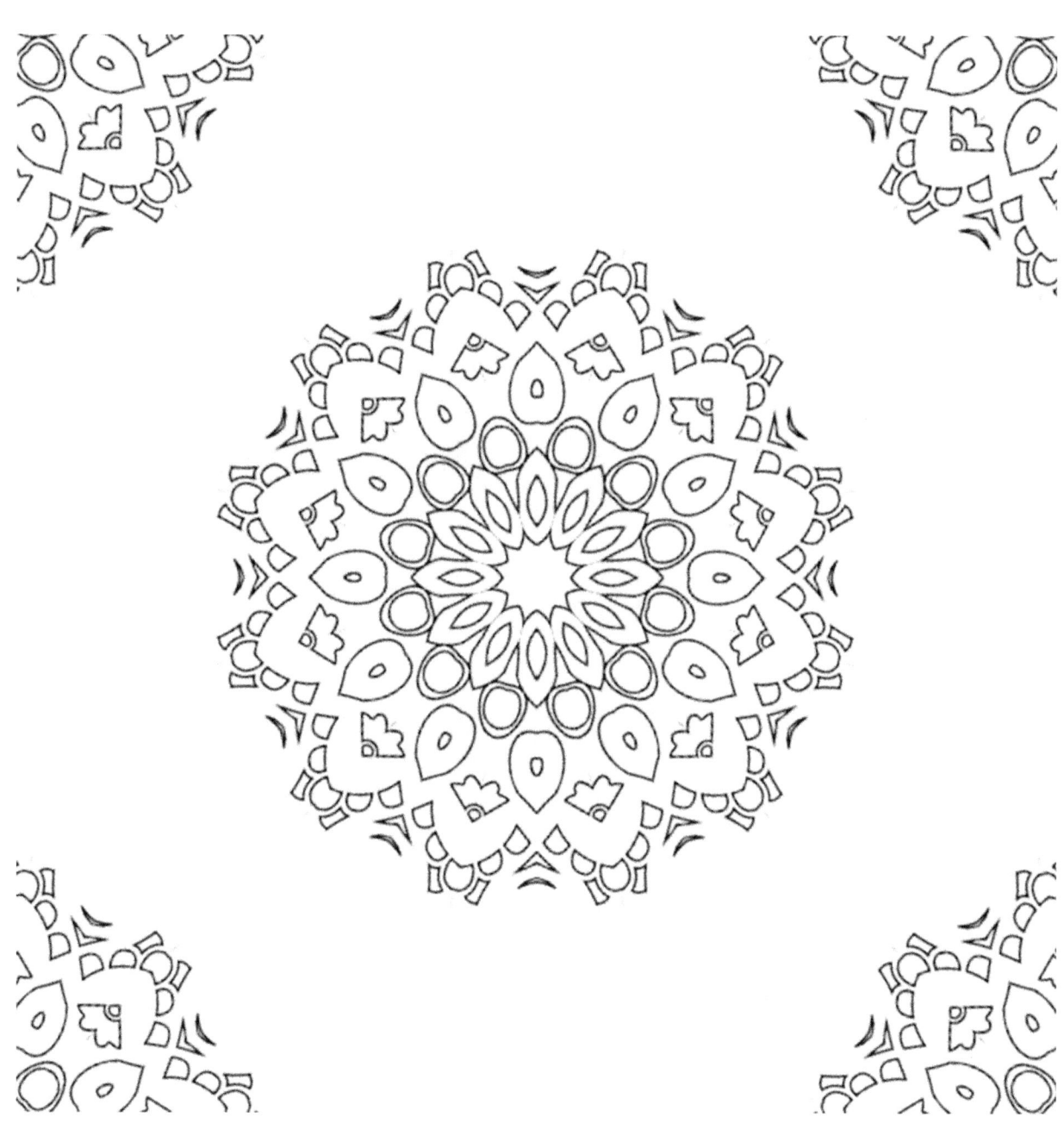

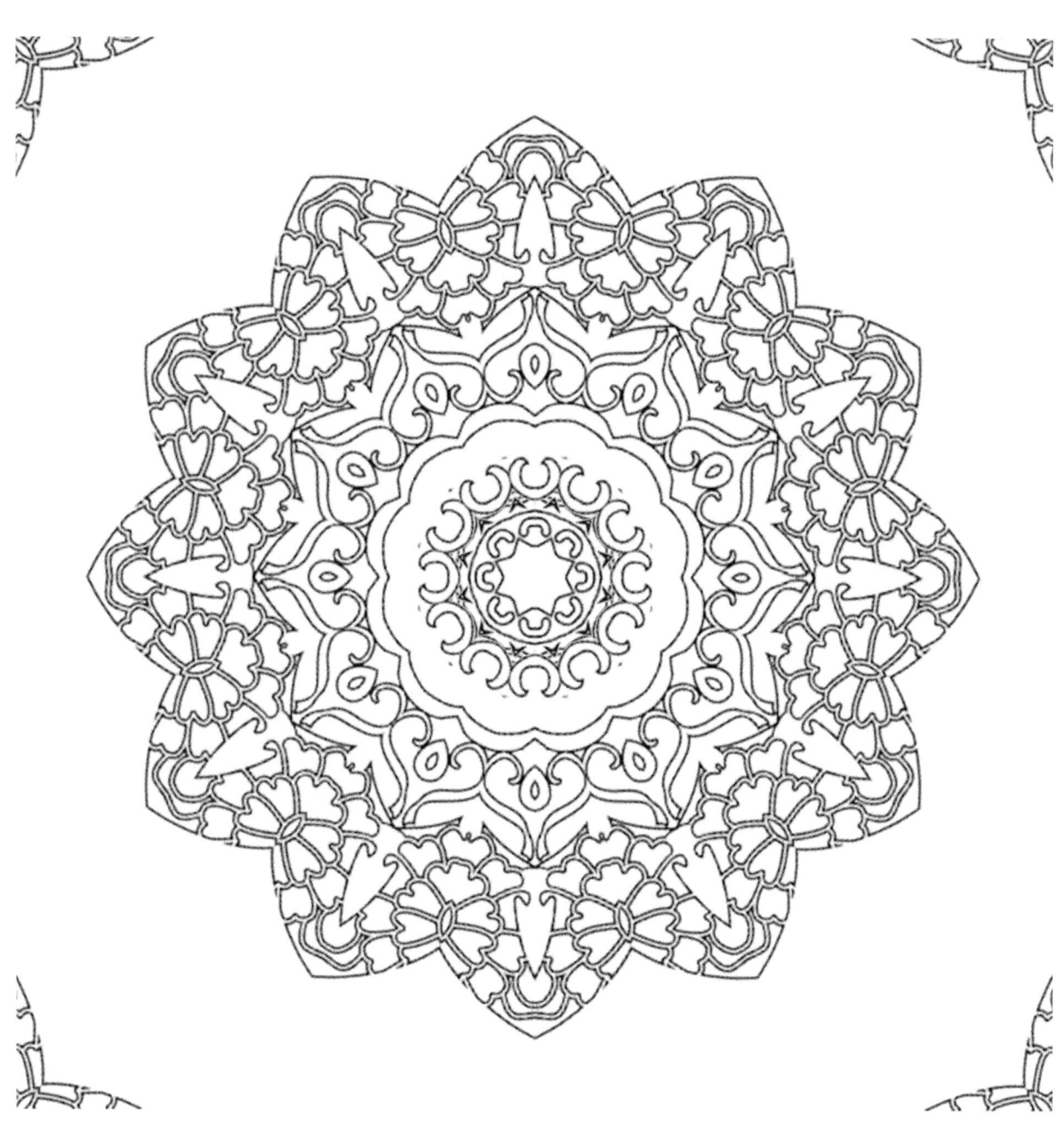

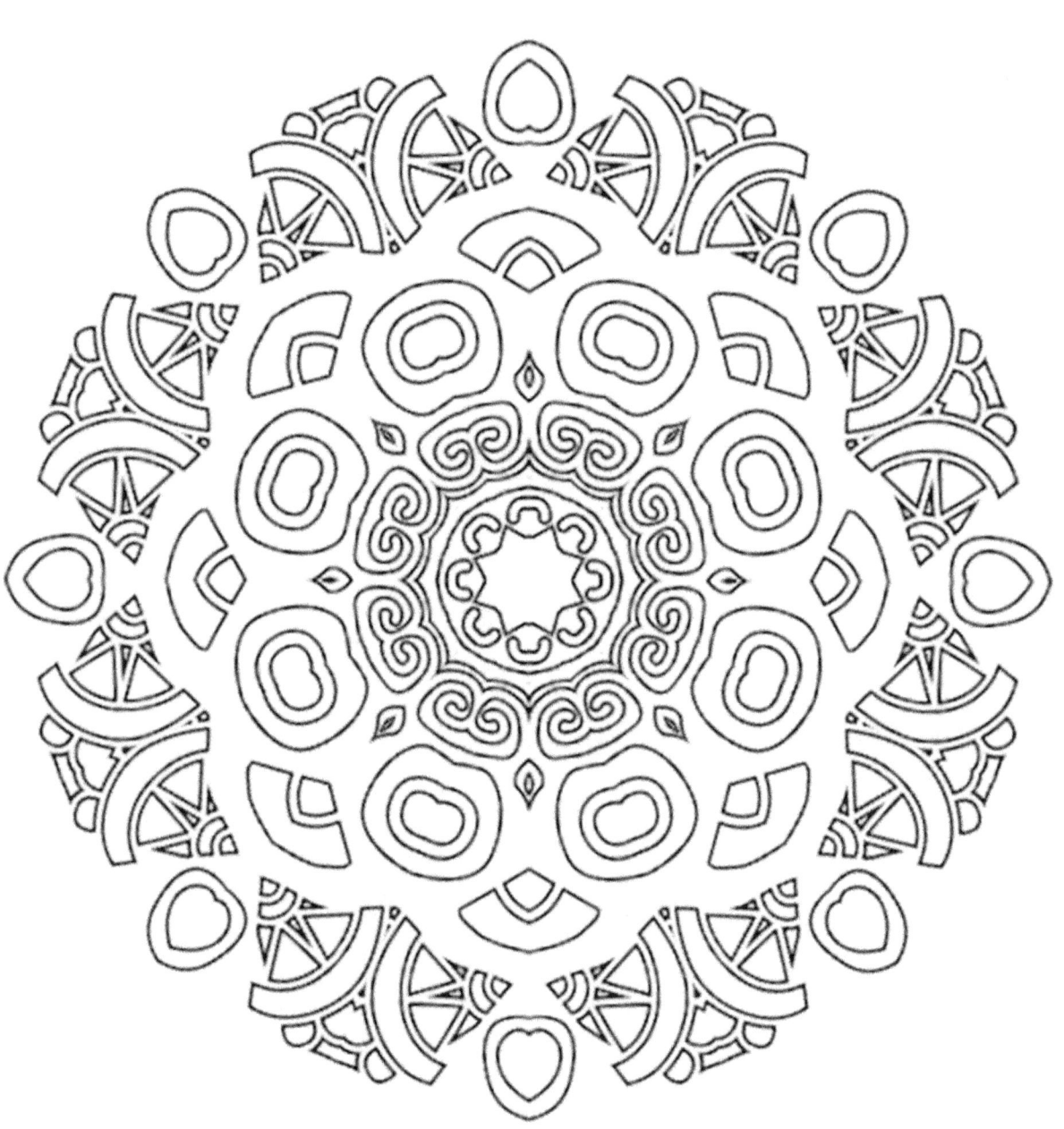

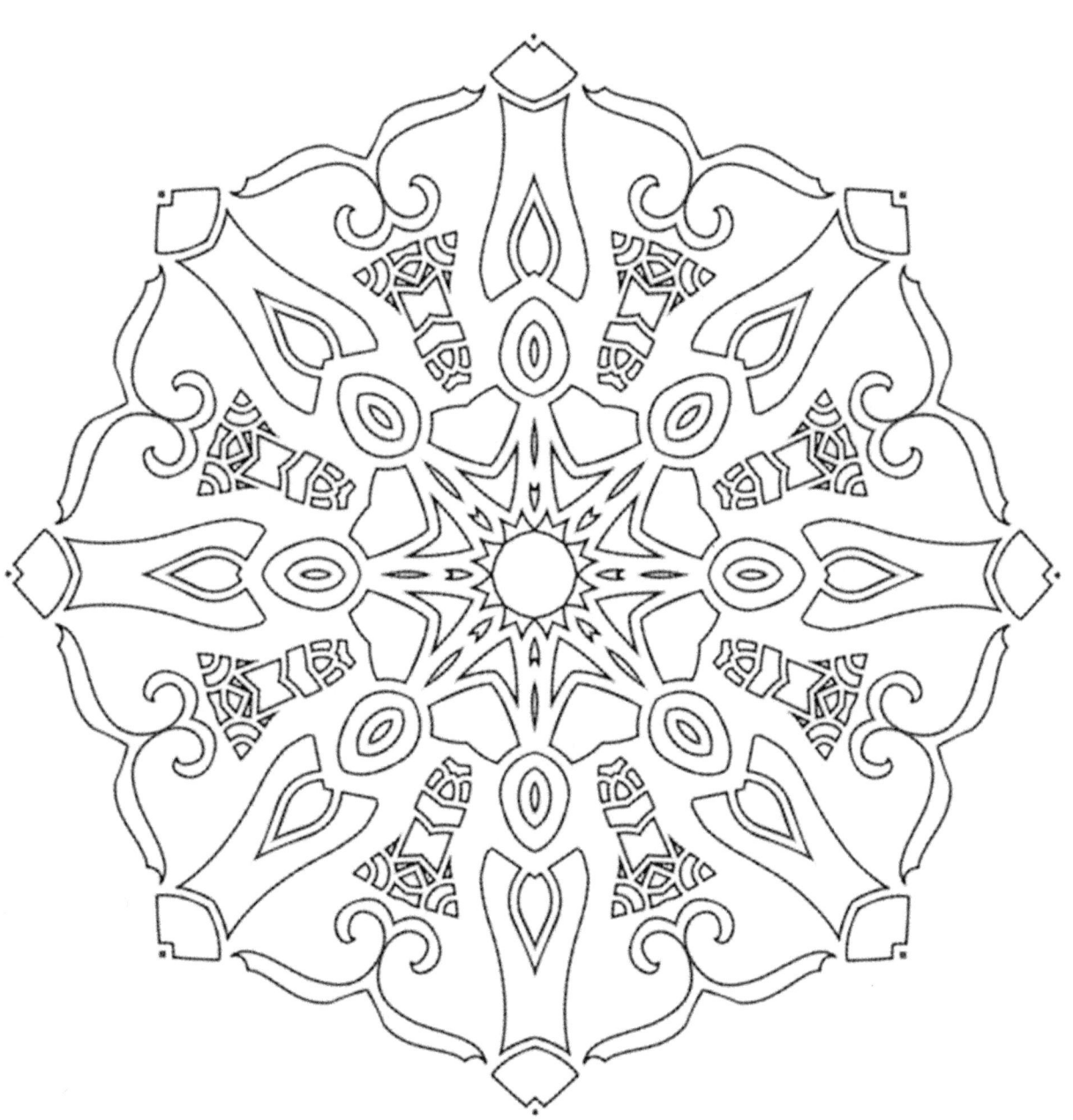

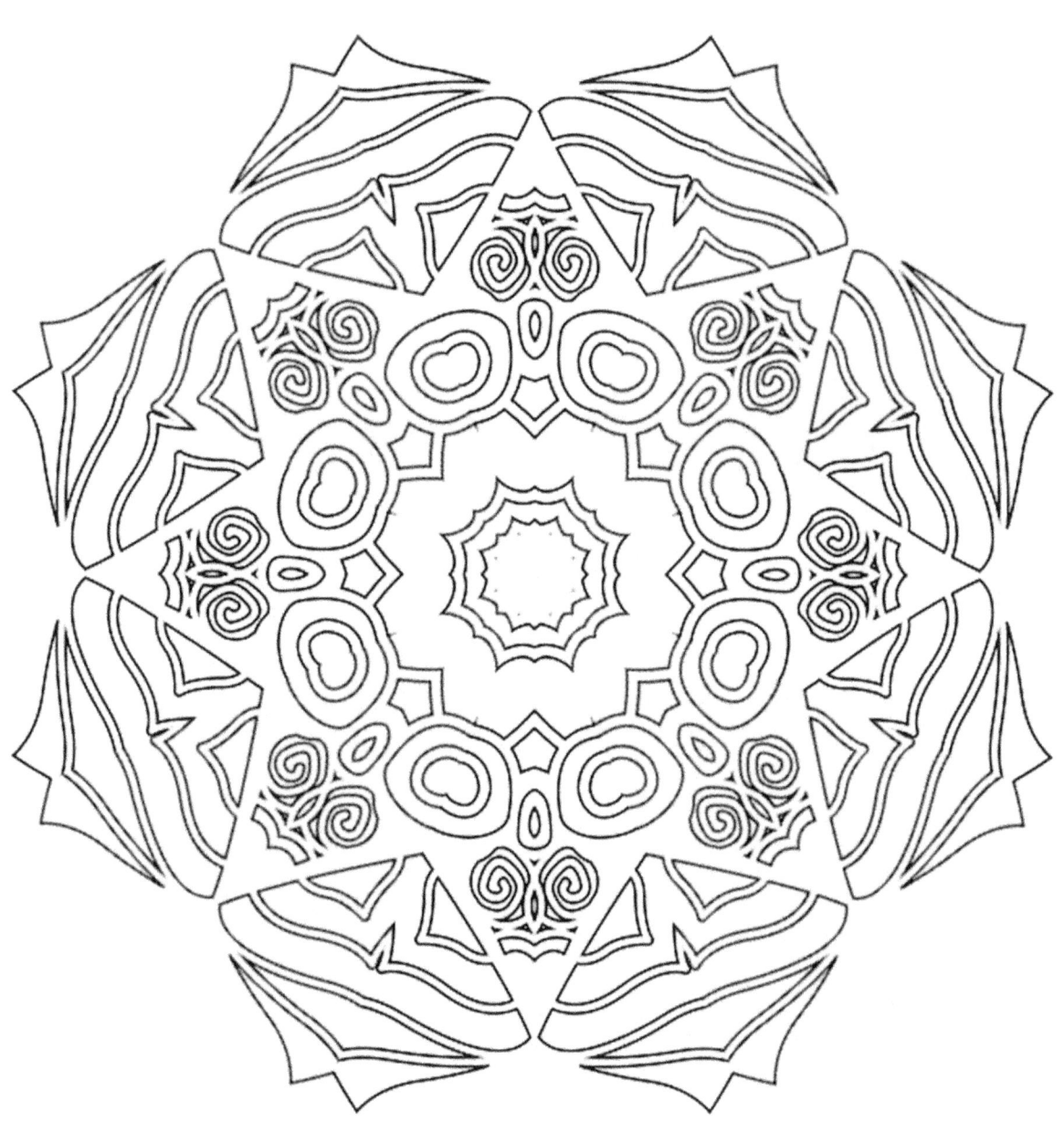

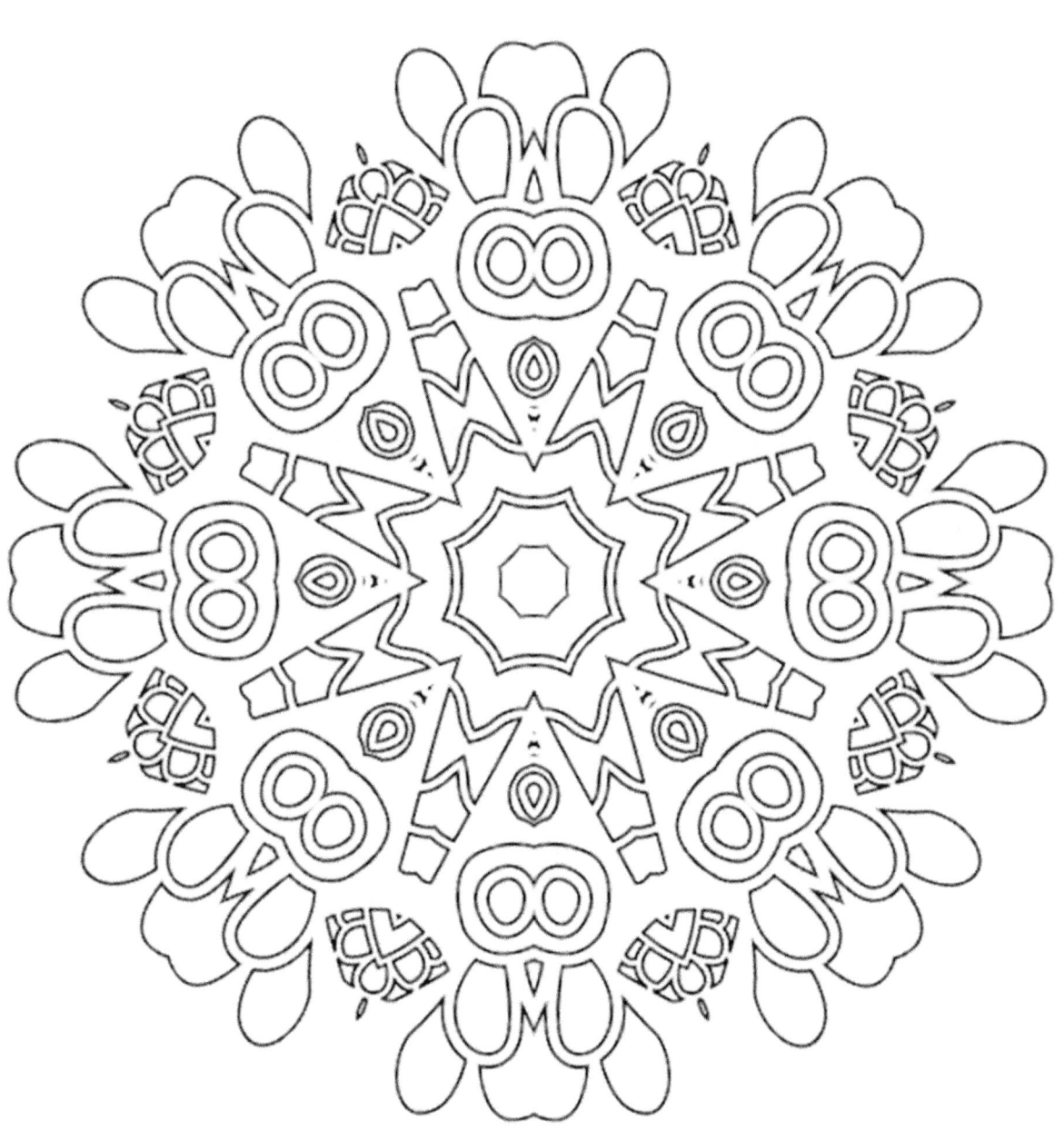

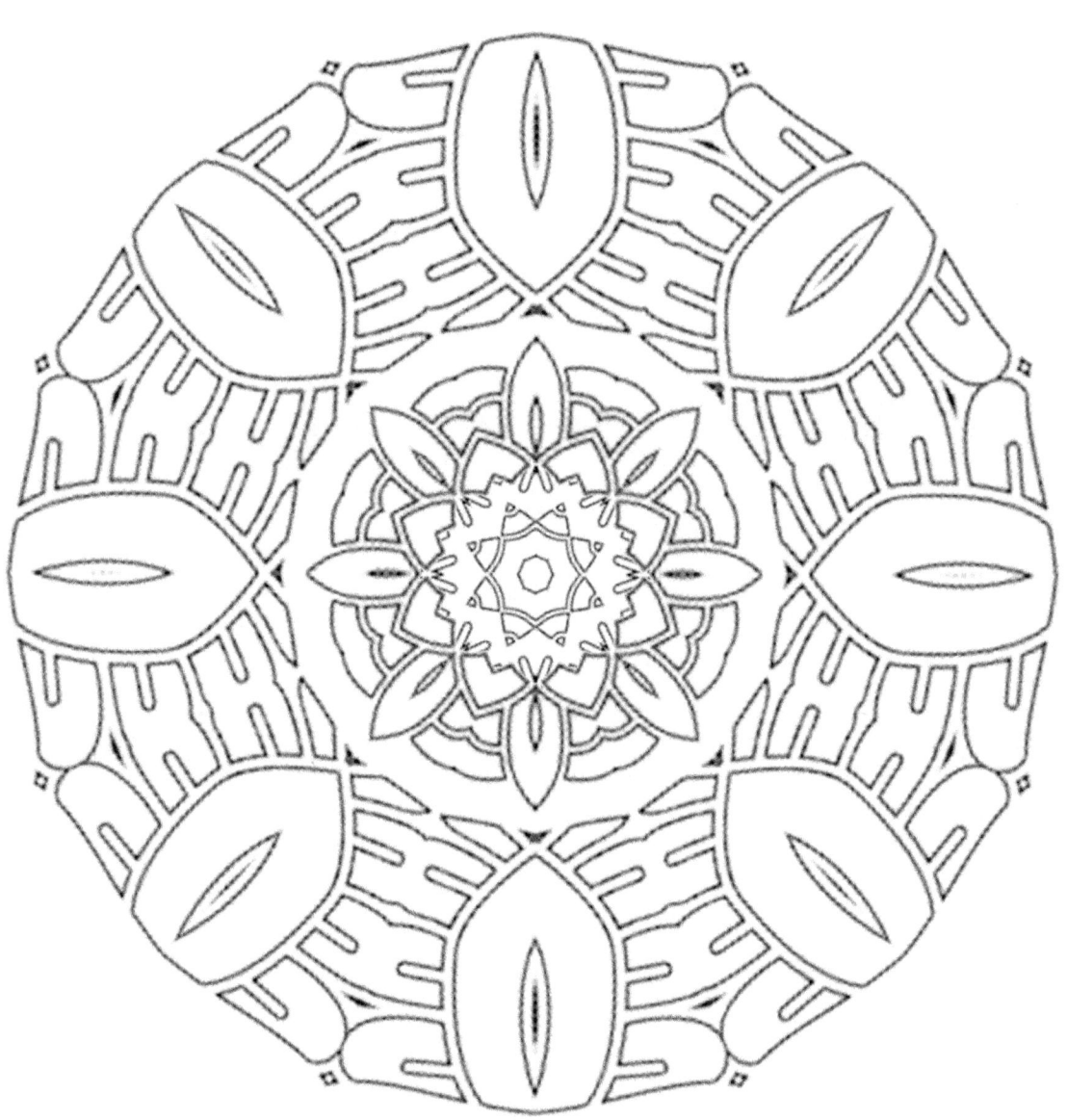

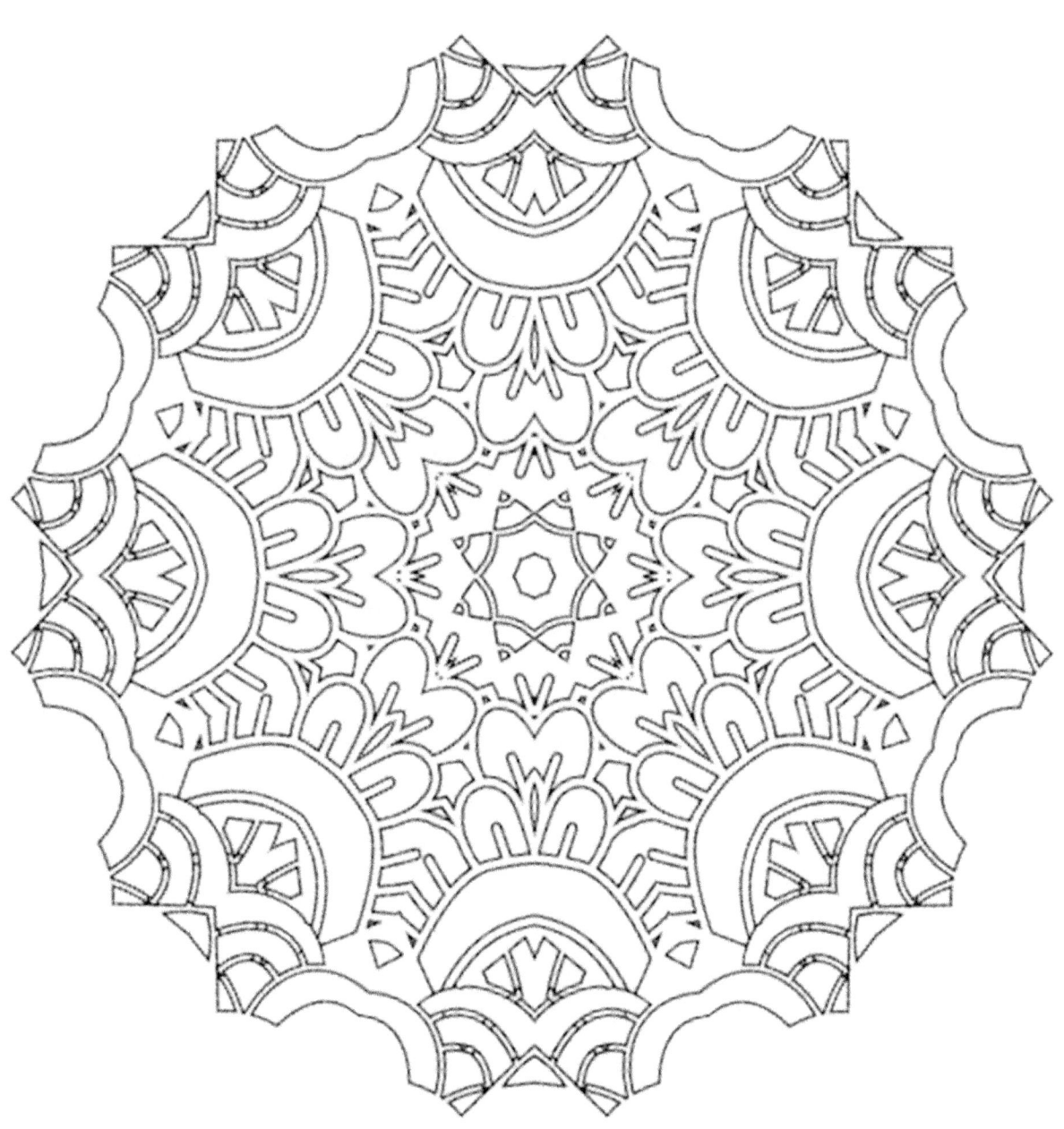

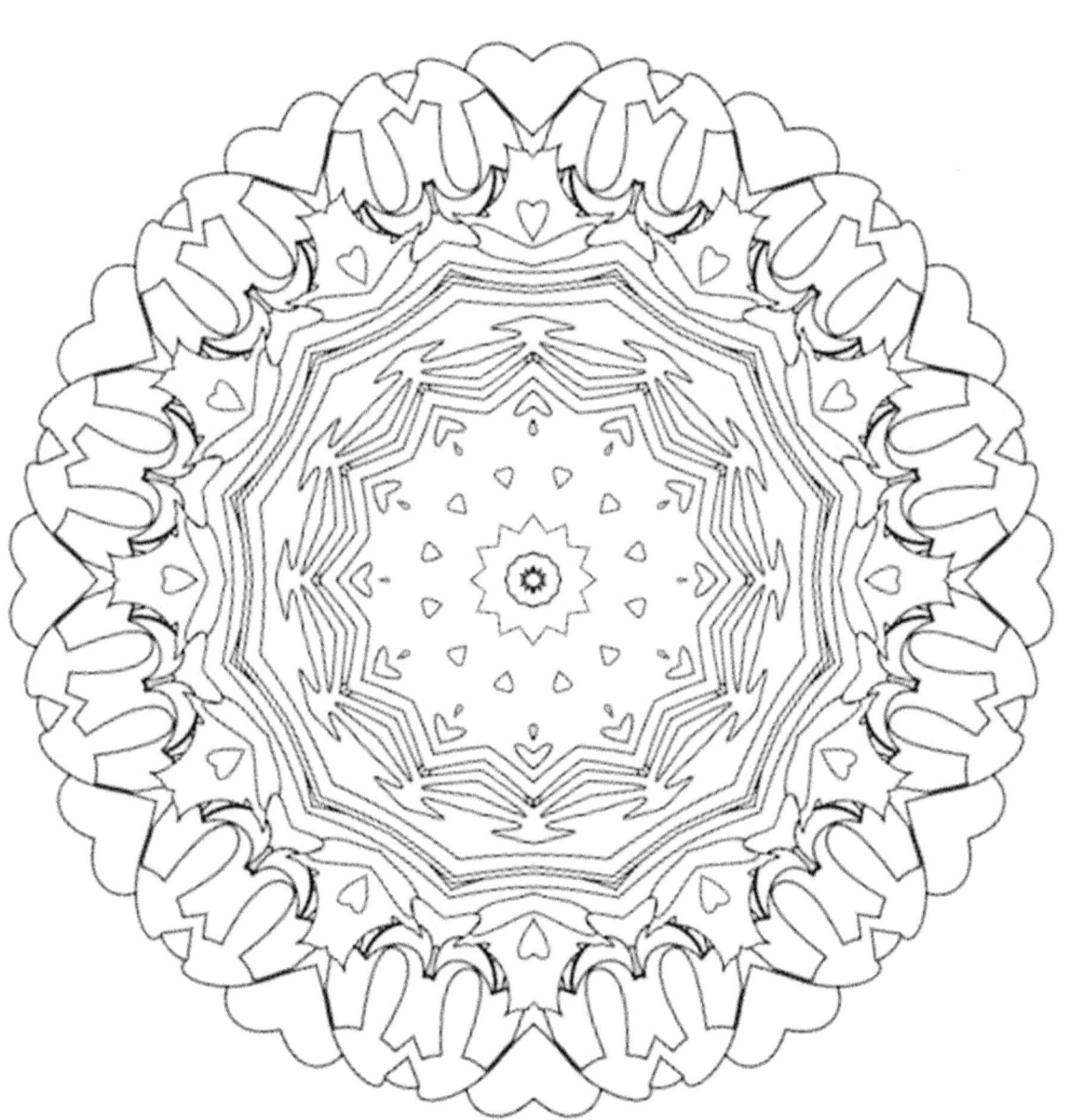

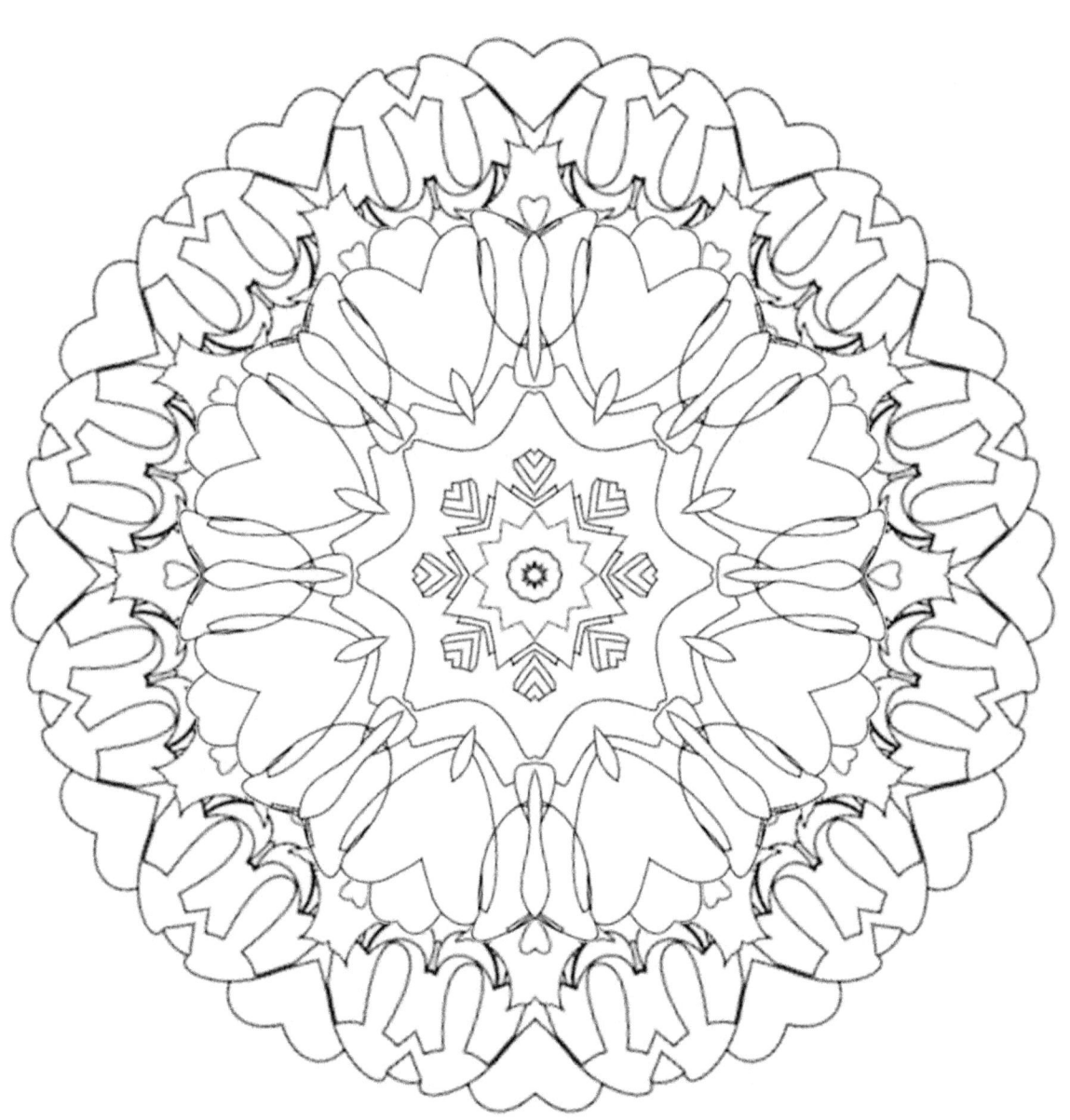

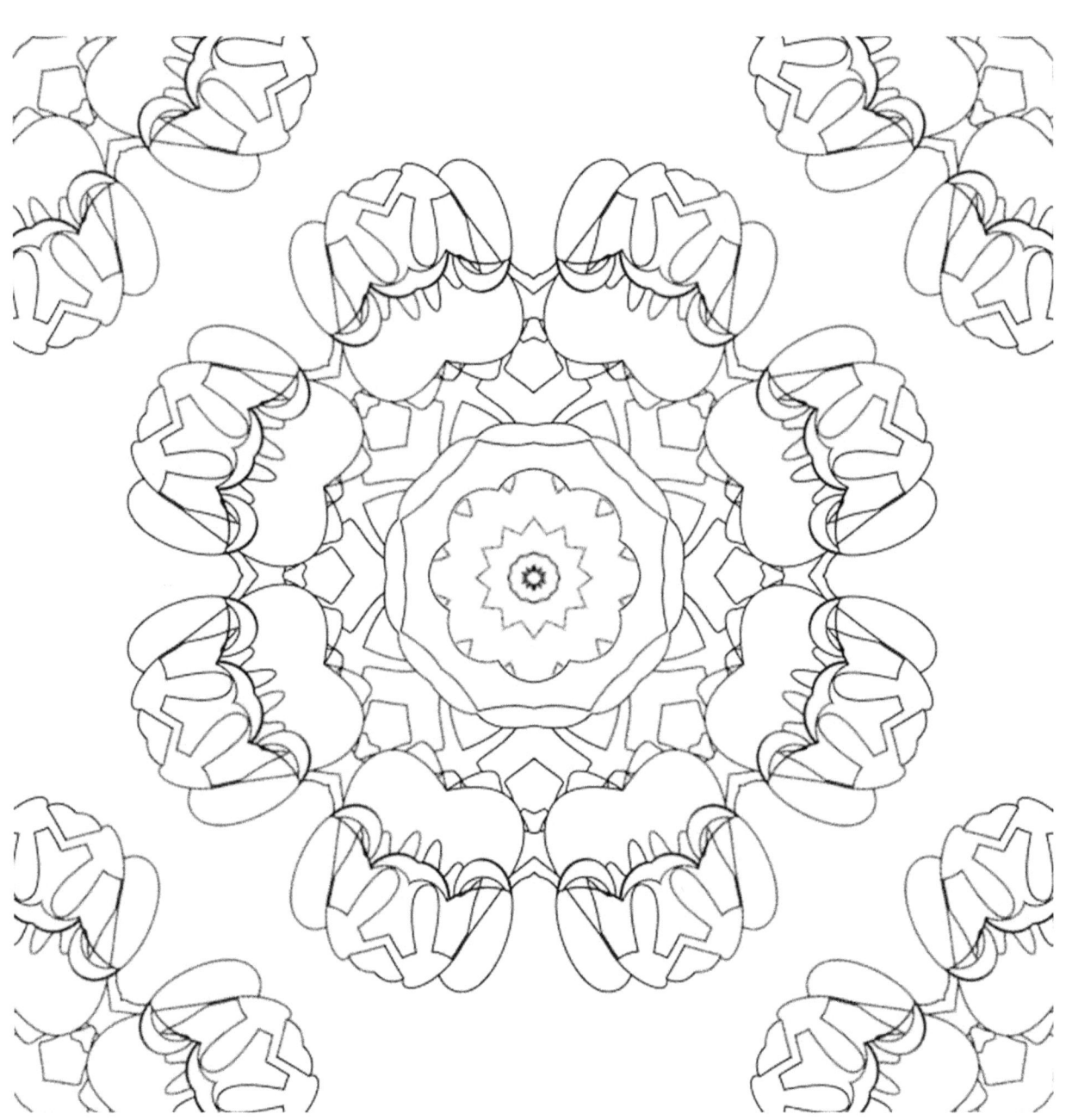

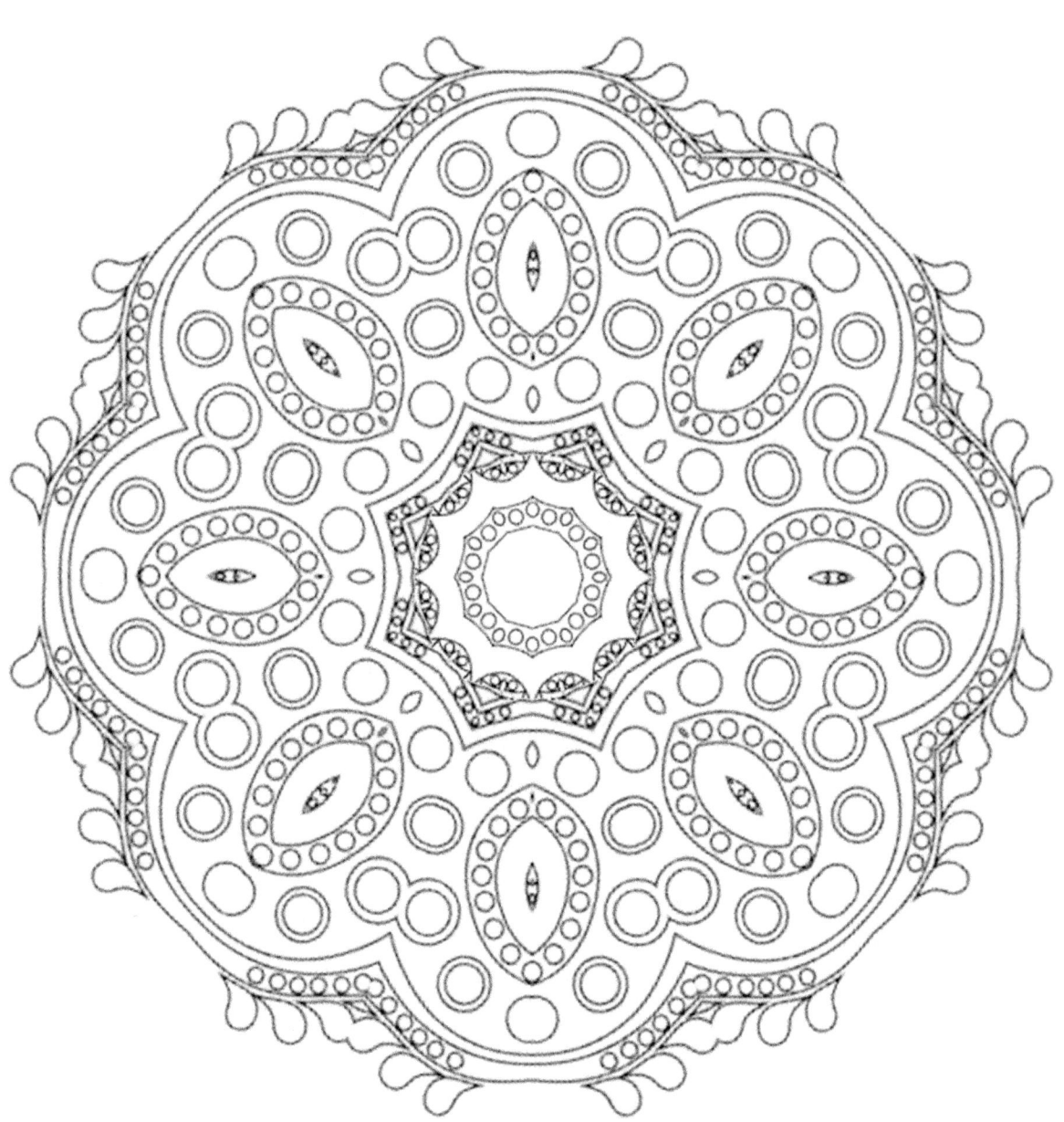

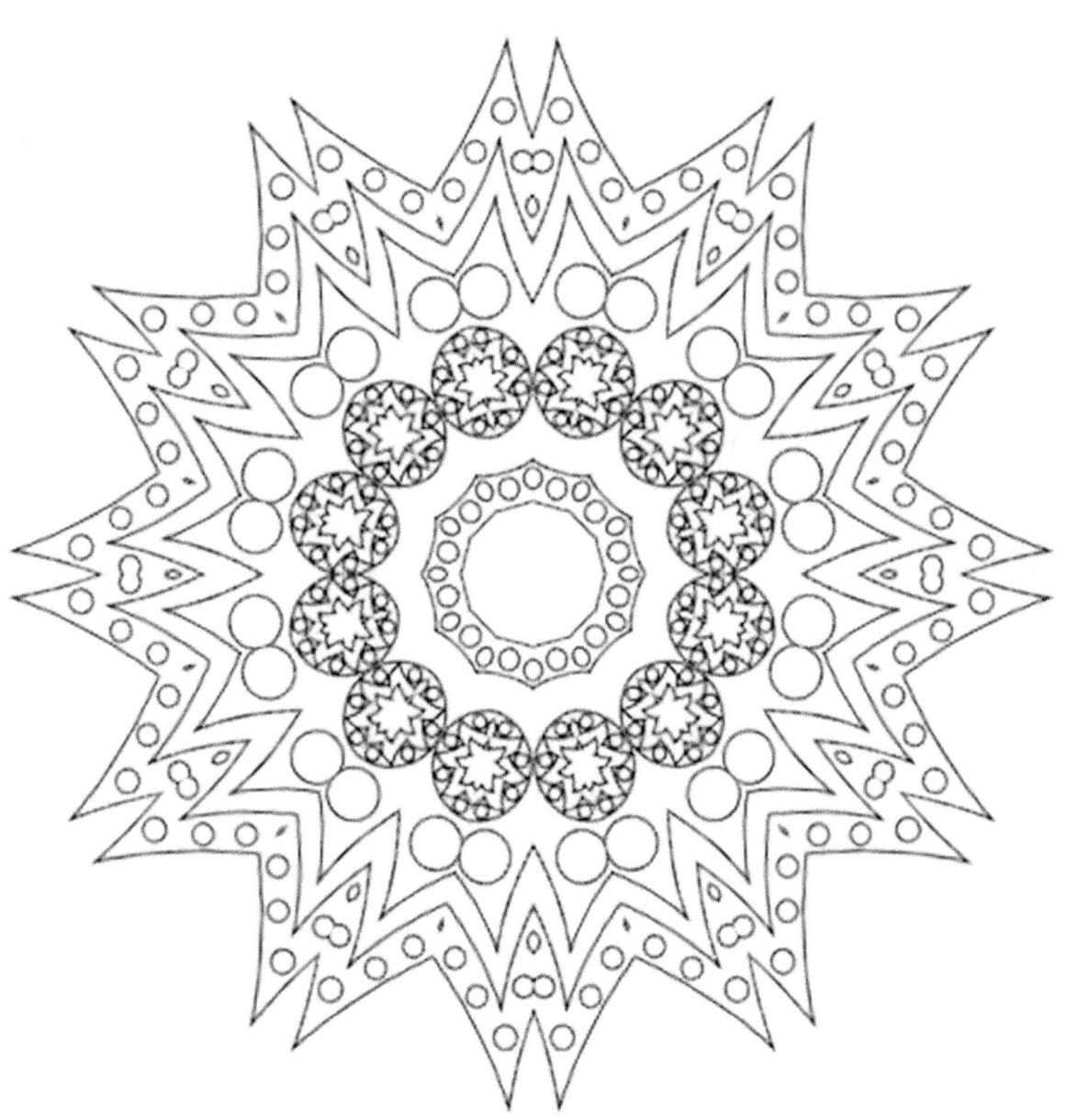

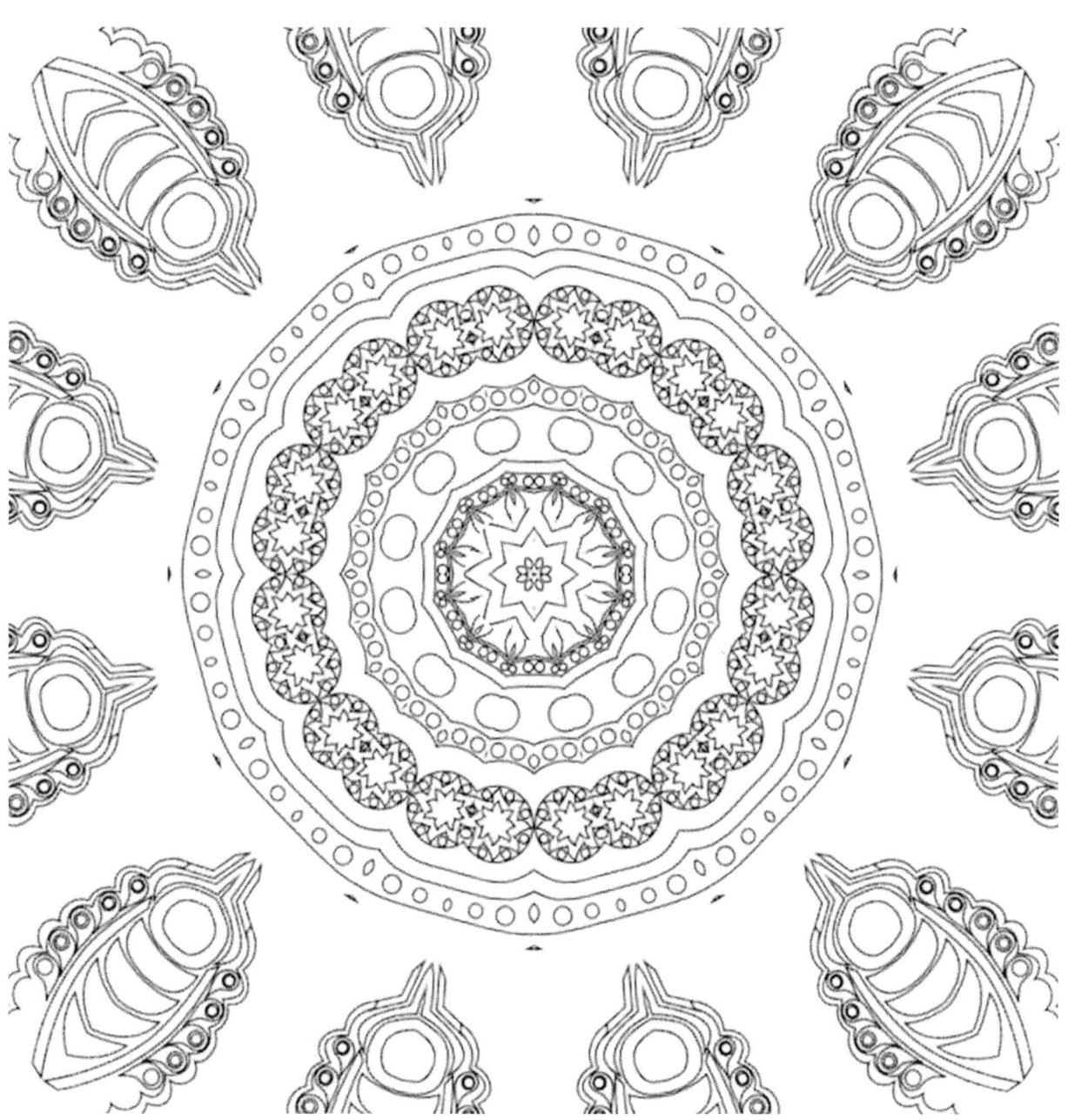

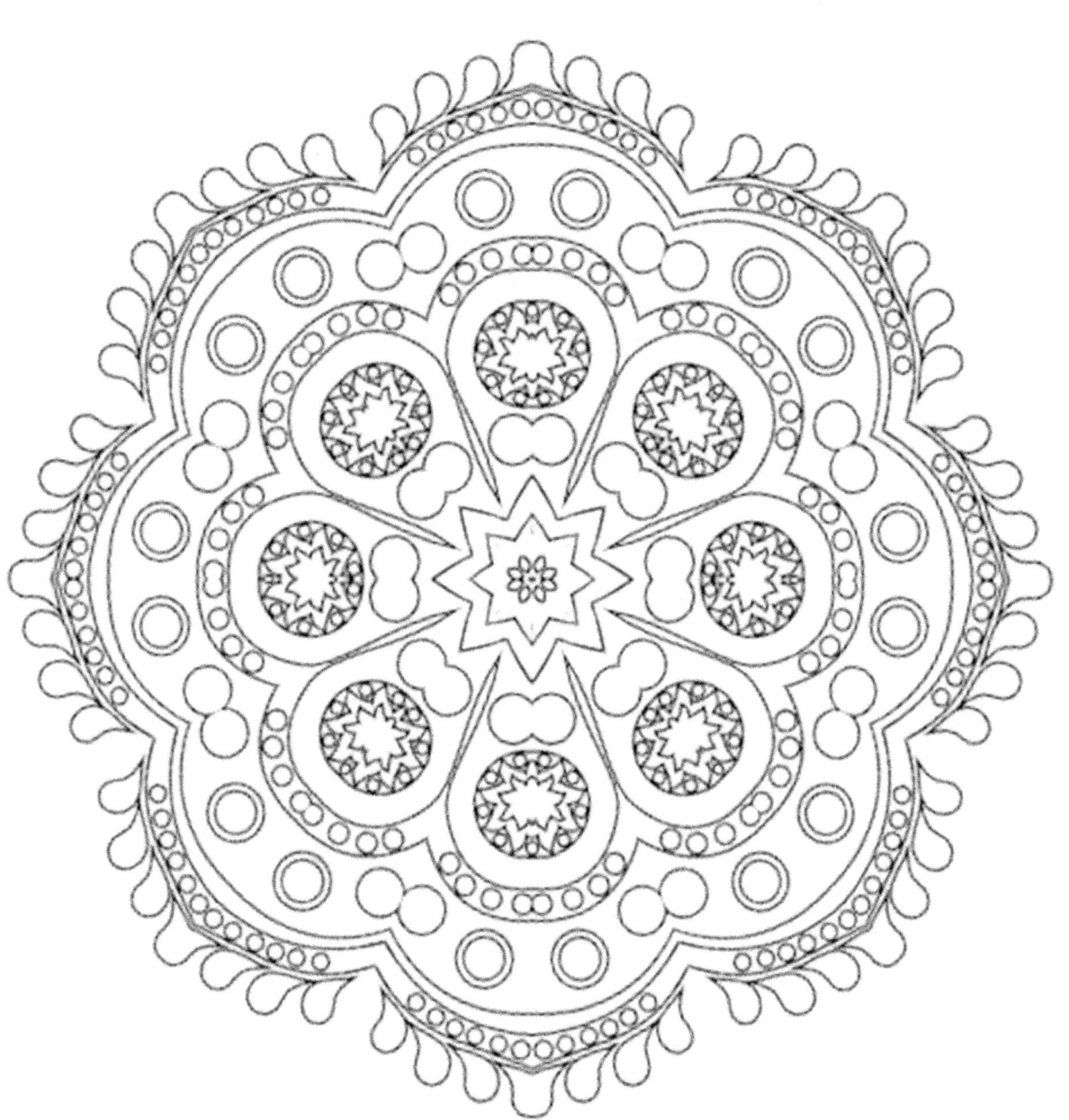

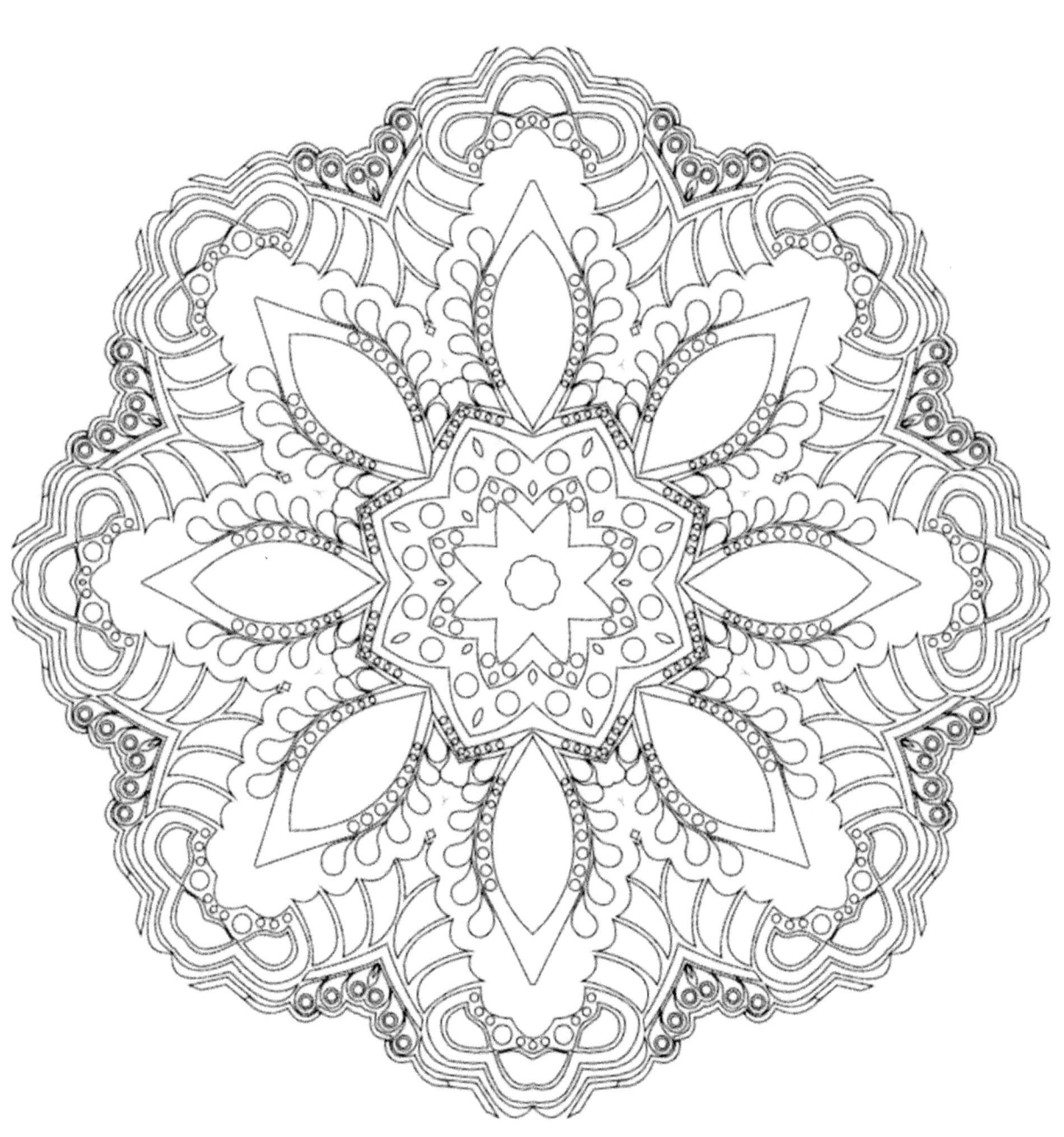

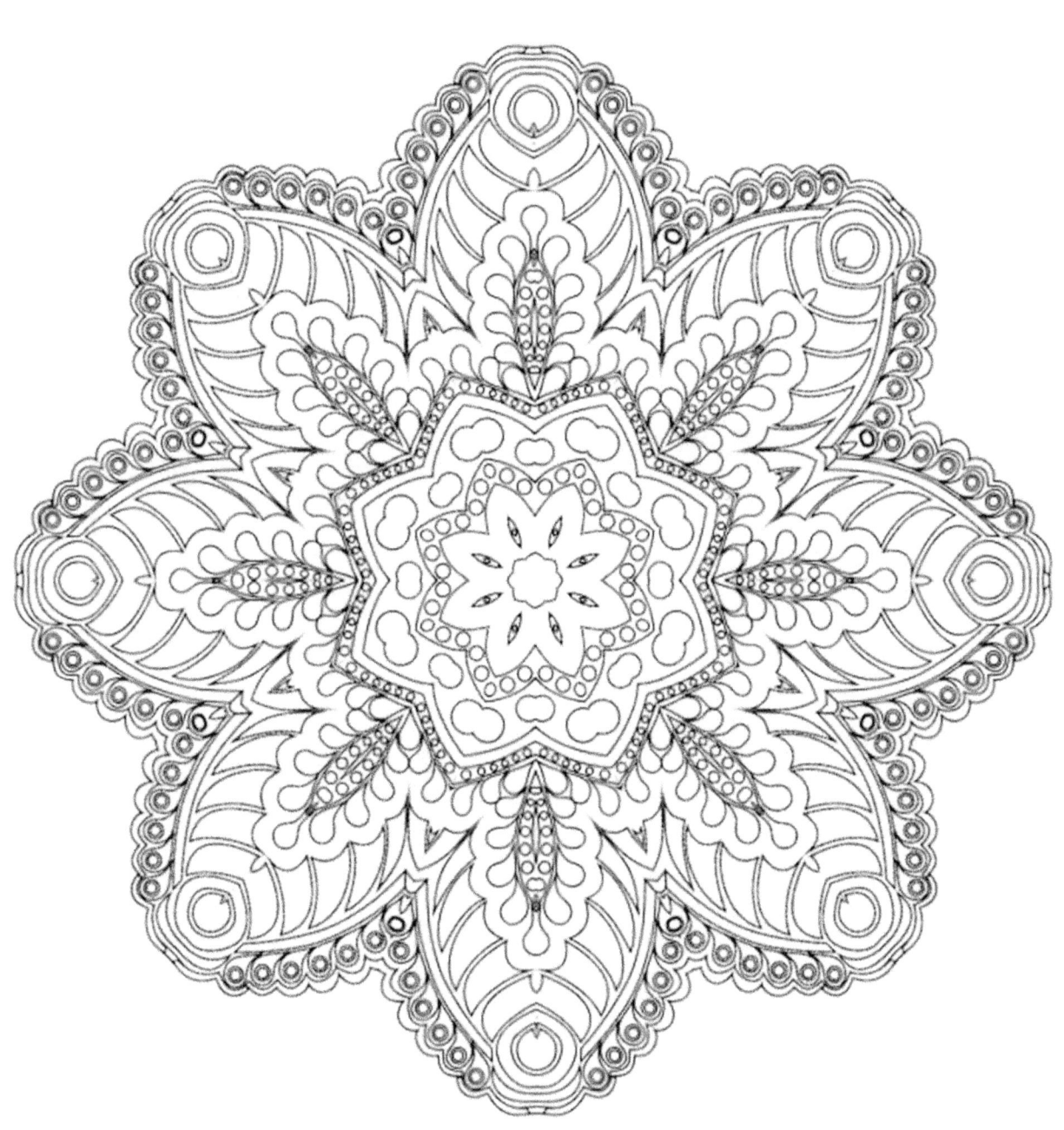

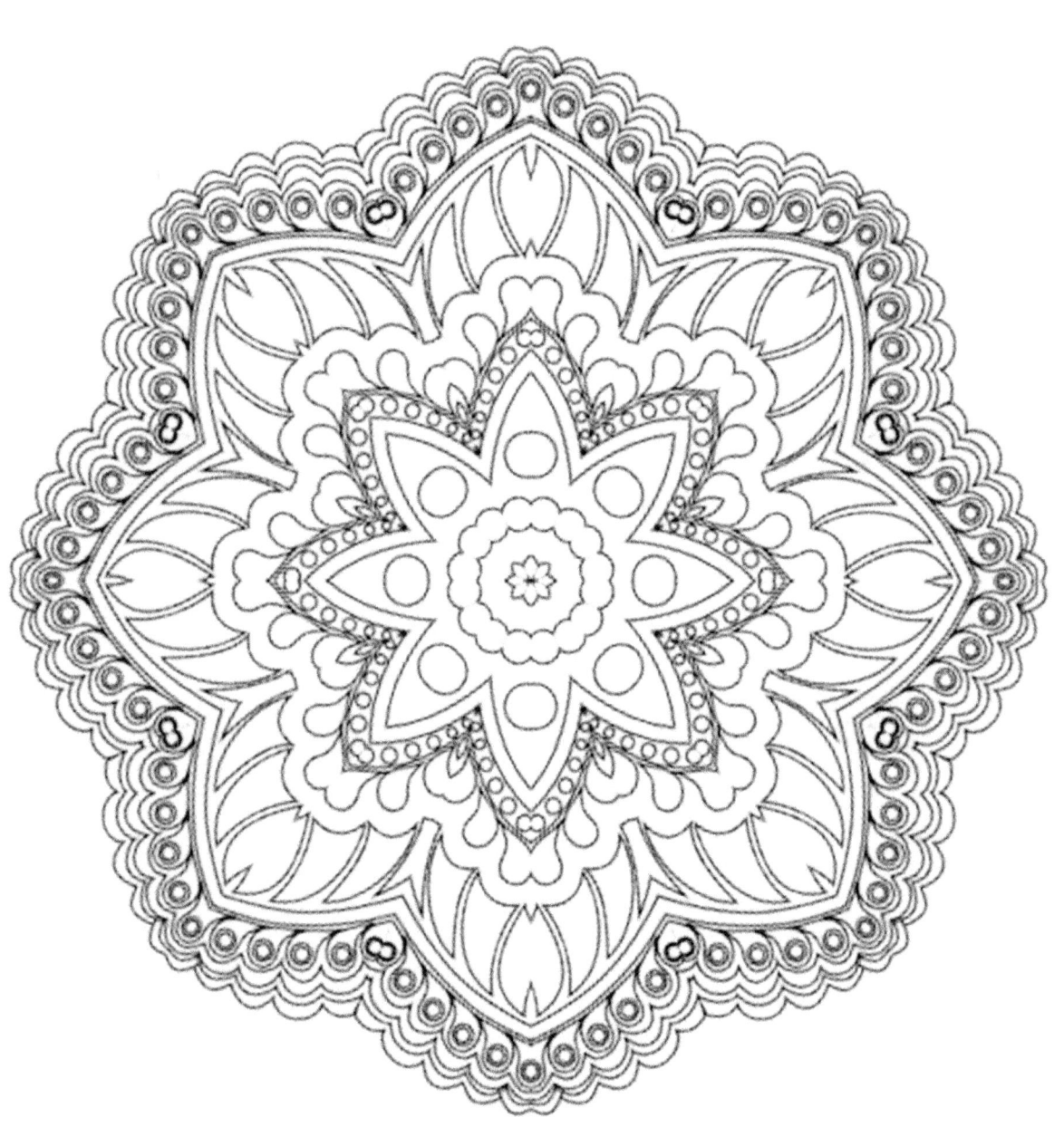

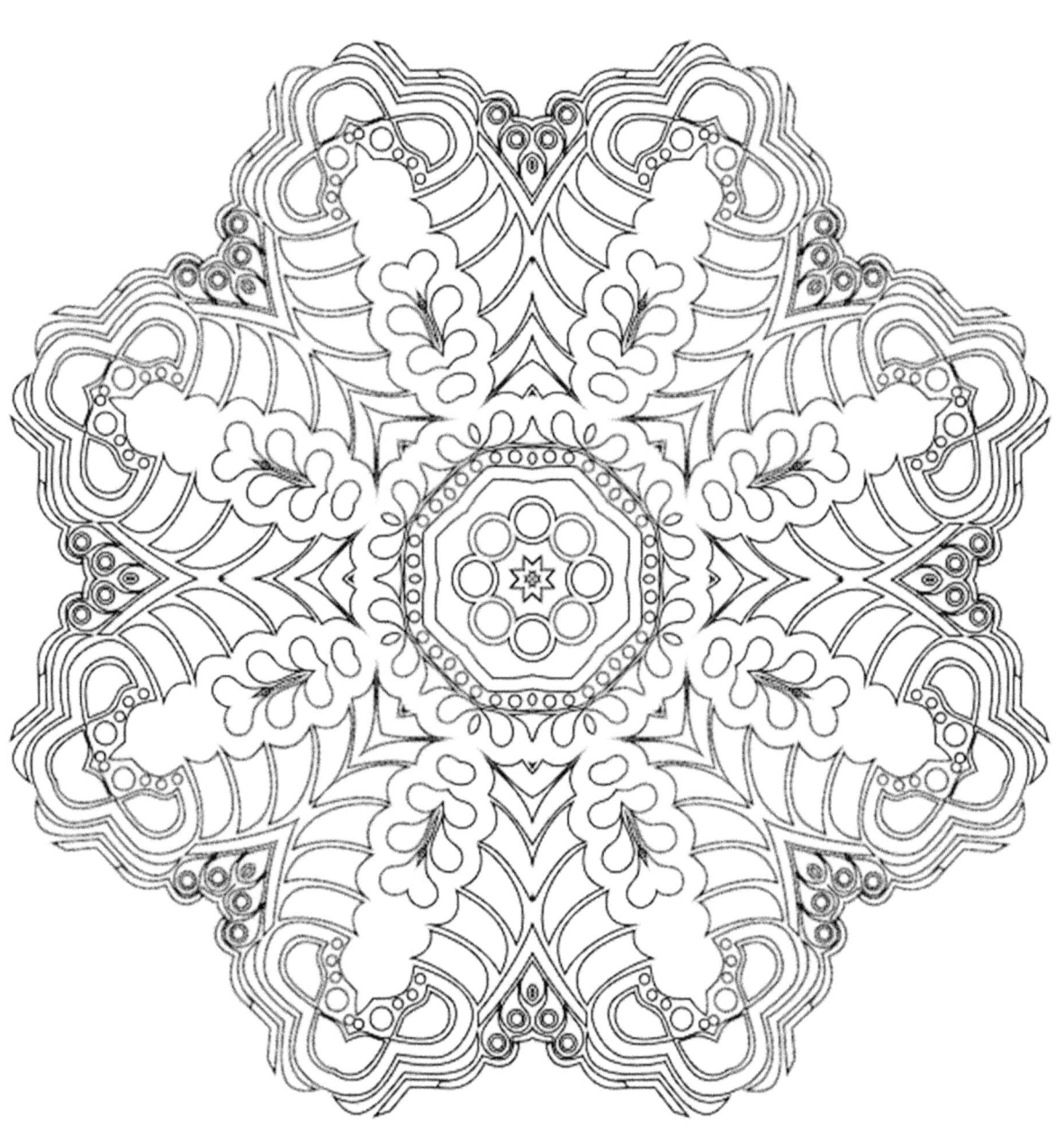

www.ingramcontent.com/pod-product-compliance
Lightning Source LLC
Chambersburg PA
CBHW080553190526
45169CB00007B/2754